Sensei Self Development

Mental Health Chronicles Series

How to Cultivate a Positive Mindset

Sensei Paul David

Copyright Page

Sensei Self Development -
How to Cultivate a Positive Mindset,
by Sensei Paul David

Copyright © 2023

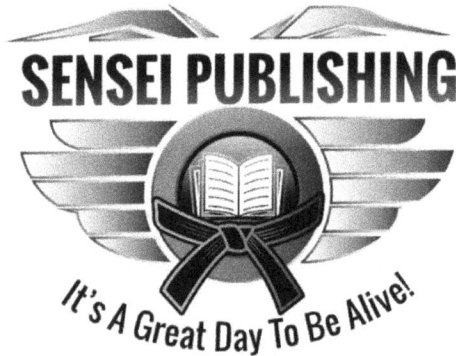

SENSEI PUBLISHING

It's A Great Day To Be Alive!

www.senseipublishing.com

@senseipublishing
#senseipublishing

Get/Share Your FREE SSD Mental Health Chronicles at
www.senseiselfdevelopment.care

or

CLICK HERE

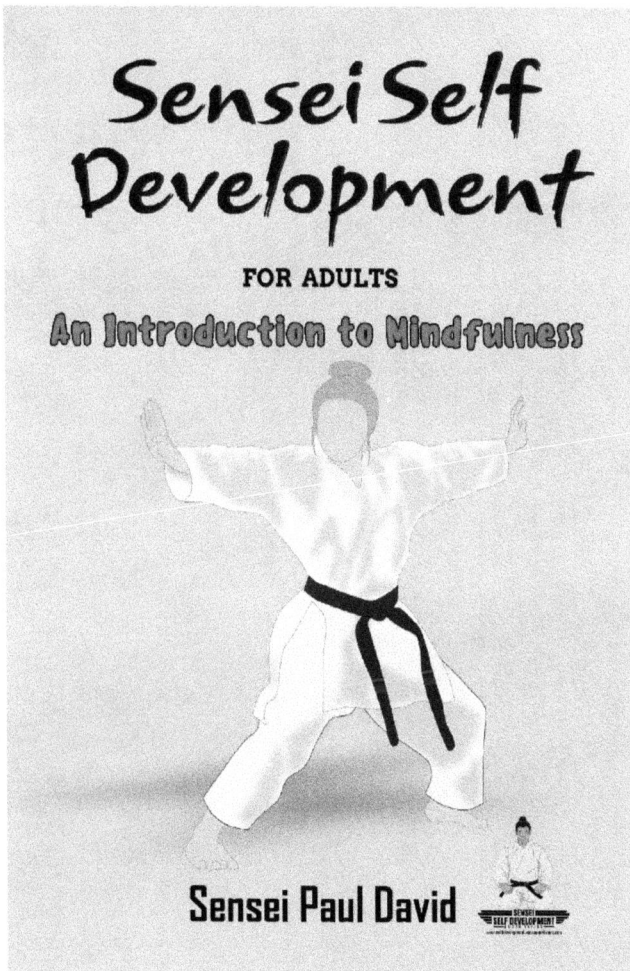

Sensei Self Development

FOR ADULTS

An Introduction to Mindfulness

Sensei Paul David

Check Out The SSD Chronicles Series CLICK HERE

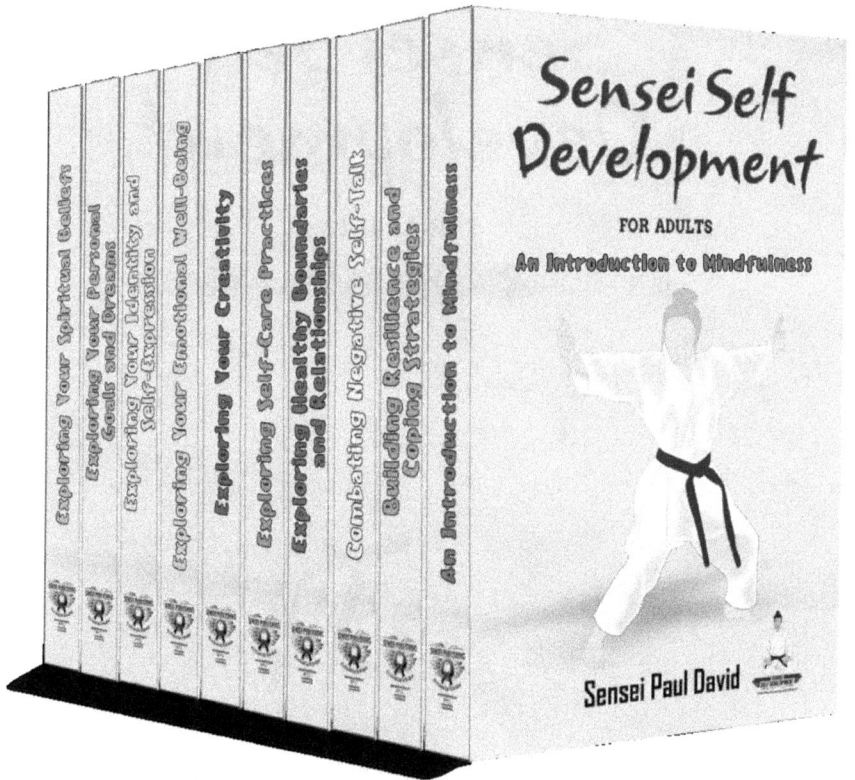

Exploring Your Spiritual Beliefs

Exploring Your Personal Goals and Dreams

Exploring Your Identity and Self-Expression

Exploring Your Emotional Well-Being

Exploring Your Creativity

Exploring Self-Care Practices

Exploring Healthy Boundaries and Relationships

Combatting Negative Self-Talk

Building Resilience and Coping Strategies

An Introduction to Mindfulness

Sensei Self Development

FOR ADULTS

An Introduction to Mindfulness

Sensei Paul David

Dedication

To those who courageously take action towards self-improvement - you are helping to evolve the world for generations to come.

- It's a great day to be alive!

If Found Please Contact:

_____

Reward If Found:

_____

MY
COMMITMENT

I, _____

commit to writing This Sensei Self
Development Journal for at least 10 days in a
row, starting: _____

Writing this journal is valuable to me because:

_____

_____

_____

_____

_____

_____

If I finish a minimum of 10 consecutive days of
writing in this journal, I will reward myself by:

_____

_____

_____

_____

_____

_____

If I don't finish 10 days of writing this journal, I will promise to:

_____

_____

_____

_____

_____

I will do the following things to ensure that I write in my Sensei Self Development Journal every day:

_____

_____

_____

_____

_____

Get/Share Your FREE All-Ages Mental Health eBook Now at
www.senseiselfdevelopment.com
Or CLICK HERE

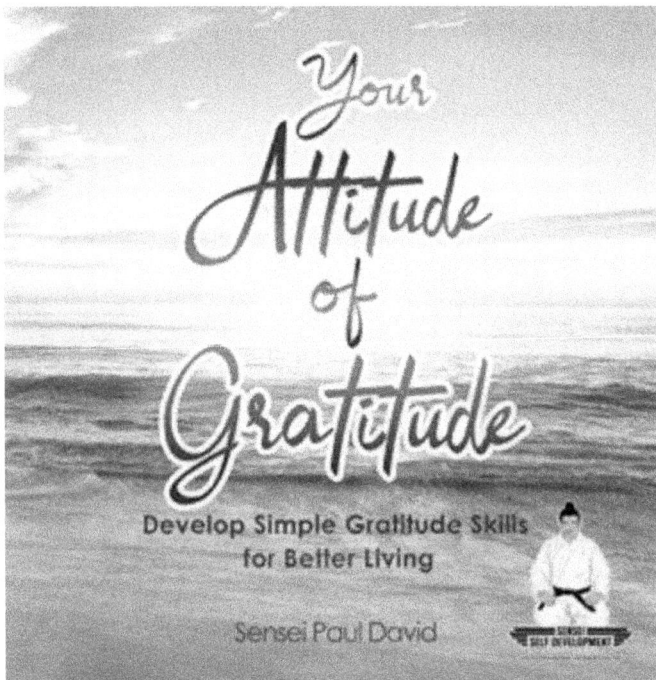

senseiselfdevelopment.com

Check Out Another Book In The
SSD BOOK SERIES:

senseipublishing.com/SSD_SERIES

CLICK HERE

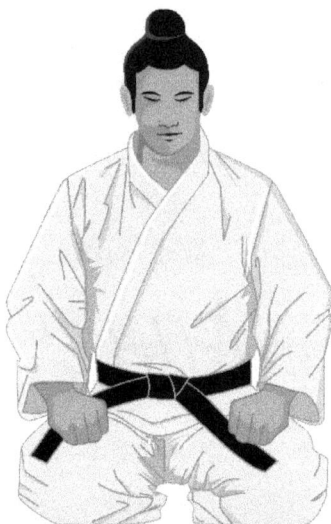

SENSEI
SELF DEVELOPMENT
BOOKS SERIES

senseiselfdevelopment.senseipublishing.com

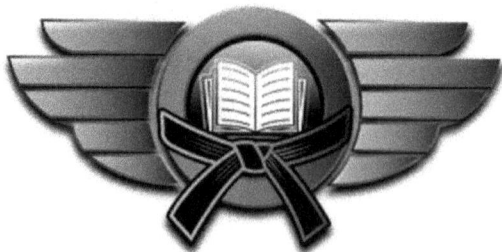

Join Our Publishing Journey!

If you would like to receive FUTURE FREE BOOKS and get to know us better, please click www.senseipublishing.com and join our newsletter by entering your email address in the pop-up box.

Follow Our Blog: senseipauldavid.ca

Follow/Like/Subscribe: Facebook, Instagram, YouTube: @senseipublishing

Scan the QR Code with your phone or tablet

to follow us on social media: Like / Subscribe / Follow

A Message From The Author:
Sensei Paul David

Dear Reader,

Welcome to the world of mental health journaling – a sacred space for self-reflection, growth, and healing. Within these pages, you hold the power to uplift your spirit, invigorate your mind, and nourish your goals.

In a world that often moves at blink-and-you'll-miss-it speed, it's crucial to make time for self-care and self-discovery.

Anxiety, stress, and emotional turbulence may have clouded your mind, making it difficult to find clarity and peace within. But fear not! Together, we will navigate the labyrinth of emotions, and experiences, helping to simplify the path to mental well-being.

This journal is not merely a bunch of blank pages awaiting your words. It is your compassionate companion, offering solace and understanding during your unique journey. Here, you are free to unburden yourself, celebrate small and large victories, and confront the challenges that may still linger.

Within the sheltered realm of these pages, there is no judgment, no expectation, and no pressure. Your unique experience and perspective hold immeasurable worth, and your voice deserves to be heard. Whether you choose to fill the lines with eloquence or simply scribble fragments of your thoughts, please remember each entry is a valuable contribution to your growth.

In this sacred space, you are challenged to take off the mask we so often wear in the outside world. It is here that you can be raw, vulnerable, and authentic – allowing your true self to be seen and embraced without reservation. By giving yourself permission to explore the depths of your emotions and confront the shadows that may lurk within, you will discover profound insights and find the healing you seek over time.

As you embark on this journaling journey, I encourage you to embrace the process itself rather than fixate solely on the outcome. Remember, it is not about reaching a certain destination or ticking off boxes on a list of accomplishments. Rather, it is about cultivating self-awareness, fostering self-compassion, and nurturing a sense of curiosity about the intricate workings of your intelligently beautiful mind.

In the quiet moments of reflection, let your pen become a bridge between your inner world and the possibilities that lie ahead. Create a sanctuary for your thoughts, fears, triumphs, and dreams. As you pour your heart onto these pages, allow your words to be a living testament to courage, resilience, and an unwavering commitment to your own well-being.

I am honored to be a part of your journey, and I believe in your ability to navigate the twists and turns with grace and resilience. Remember, you are not alone in this – countless others have walked similar paths, faced similar challenges, and emerged stronger and wiser on the other side. You have the power to reclaim all of your untapped joy, cultivate a positive mindset that serves you, and foster a deep sense of self-love and peaceful confident. – And it will take a worth effort and time.

So, open the first page of this journal with hope, curiosity, and an open heart and open mind. Embrace the transformative power of self-reflection, and allow it to guide you towards a life of greater fulfilment and peace. Each journaling session is an opportunity to not only connect with yourself but also to rekindle the light within that sometimes flickers but never extinguishes.

Remember, the pages you are about to fill are not just a record of your journey but also a testament to your strength, resilience, and indomitable spirit. Cherish this space, invest in yourself, and let your words be an ode to the magnificent journey of becoming whole.

With great respect for your decision to evolve,

Paul

MY CONVICTION

Please circle your answers below

I am DECIDING to be patient with myself and this PROCESS each time I journal toward my improved state of mental well-being

YES   NO

"The present moment is filled with joy and happiness. If you are attentive, you will see it."

Thich Nhat Hanh

Introduction

Do you find yourself looking at life through a lens of optimism or one of pessimism? The way we perceive the world shapes our experiences in it.

Take a moment to reflect: What are your thoughts about your life and its future? Do you often foresee challenges and obstacles, or do you picture a journey filled with hope and opportunities?

In our modern, fast-paced world, where negative news often dominates, maintaining a positive outlook can be a challenge. Daily life is bustling, and through media and online platforms, we're frequently exposed to narratives of negativity, scarcity, and fear. The recent pandemic and ongoing wars in Ukraine and Palestine have only intensified these feelings.

It's all too easy to slip into a negative mindset, sometimes without even noticing it. Before you know it, you might find yourself pondering when and how things started to look so bleak.

Harboring a negative outlook can cause anxiety and isolation. If past efforts to control or impact the world around you failed, you might feel even more disheartened. But there's always one significant change within your reach: transforming yourself. How? By cultivating a positive mindset.

Positive mindset is not just a feel-good mantra; it's a concept supported by science. Embracing positivity can revolutionize your attitude, behavior, and ultimately, your overall happiness.

Remember Mahatma Gandhi's words: "Keep your thoughts positive because your thoughts become your words. Keep your words positive because your words become your behavior. Keep your behavior positive because your behavior becomes your habits. Keep your habits positive because your habits become your values. Keep your values positive because your values become your destiny."

Gandhi's quote elegantly ties together the chain reaction between our thoughts, actions, and destiny. Essentially, if you cultivate positive thoughts, this optimism will seep into your speech and behavior. In turn, this influences your habits, values, and ultimately shapes your future. Sounds promising, right?

But let's break down what "Positive Mindset" means exactly.

Positive mindset isn't about ignoring life's challenges or pretending they don't exist. It's not a call for naivety or turning a blind eye to problems. Rather, it's about confronting unpleasant situations with a positive and productive mindset, rooted in logic and reason. It's neither about always expecting the worst nor maintaining an irrational, unwavering positivity.

Building a positive mindset begins with how you talk to yourself and how you perceive the world around you. It's about self-reflection and a reasoned understanding of your environment.

Psychologist describes positive thinking as:

- Facing challenges with optimism;
- Finding the silver lining in tough situations;
- Seeing the best in others;
- Having a positive view of oneself and one's abilities.

So, now that we've unpacked the concept of a positive mindset, you might wonder why it's beneficial. What do you gain from shifting your attitude? Let's explore that.

Benefits of Positive Mindset

Positive Mindset and Physical Health

"In a garden of weeds, be a wildflower."

"The night is darkest just before dawn."

"A smooth sea never made a skilled sailor"

"A joyful heart sees a festive world,"

"Keep your face towards the sunshine and the shadows will fall behind you,"

Researchers are finding that these kinds of optimistic perspectives do more than just brighten our mood – they can significantly enhance our health and even extend our lifespan.

The connection between our mental state and physical well-being is increasingly evident. In times of health crises, nurturing positive emotions can strengthen the immune system and ward off depression. Numerous studies have shown a clear link between a positive outlook and various health benefits, such as lower blood pressure, reduced risk of heart disease, better weight control, and healthier blood sugar levels.

For instance, a study by the Harvard School of Public Health observed over 70,000 women over eight years. They found that those with a more optimistic outlook had a notably lower risk (almost 30% less) of dying from heart-related conditions. Published in the American Journal of Epidemiology, this research suggests that maintaining a positive mindset could be key in reducing heart disease risk.

Another significant study in the journal Psychosomatic Medicine investigated the relationship between positive emotions and the body's immune response. In this experiment, volunteers were exposed to a common cold virus. Remarkably, those who reported more frequent positive emotions were less likely to catch the cold. This study offers strong evidence that a positive mindset can bolster our immune system, making it more effective against infections.

These insights remind us that keeping "your face always toward the sunshine" can truly cause the "shadows to fall behind you," not just in spirit but also in health.

Positive Mindset and Negative Emotions

Psychology has witnessed a significant evolution over the past two decades. For a long time, the primary focus was on diminishing negative emotions like anxiety, stress, and depression. The goal was to help individuals move up from deeply negative states, say from a -5 to a -1 on an emotional scale, essentially reducing their level of misery.

However, the last two decades have seen a paradigm shift with the advent of positive psychology. This new branch of psychology places a spotlight on cultivating positive thoughts and behaviors, aiming not just to alleviate misery but to actively foster happiness and well-being.

What's interesting is that research in this area has shown that increasing positive emotions doesn't just make people happier; it also contributes to diminishing negative feelings. It turns out that enhancing positive emotions can be a powerful method in lessening misery.

A pivotal figure in this field is Martin Seligman, often referred to as the father of modern positive psychology. In a series of studies he conducted over the years, Seligman explored the impact of positive psychology interventions. These interventions, designed to boost positive emotions, were found to not only elevate levels of happiness in participants but also significantly reduce symptoms of depression.

Positive Mindset and Resilience

Resilient individuals, those who bounce back from adversity, often share a common trait: they tend to view difficulties as temporary and manageable. This doesn't mean they ignore problems or pretend everything is fine when it's not. Instead, they approach obstacles with a sense of hope and the belief that they can find a way through. Their positive outlook enables them to see setbacks as opportunities for growth and learning, rather than insurmountable roadblocks. This attitude helps them recover from setbacks more quickly and with less distress, demonstrating the tangible benefits of a positive mindset in building resilience.

In a study published in Nature, with older adults, positive thinking training was found to significantly boost resilience. The training involved weekly sessions for two months, teaching positive thinking strategies. Participants showed a marked increase in their ability to cope with life's challenges, demonstrating that positive thinking can play a key role in enhancing resilience among the elderly.

Positive Mindset and Performance

Research has shown that when people adopt a positive mindset at work, they tend to see improvements in pretty much everything – from how much they get done (productivity), to their originality (creativity), to how invested they are in their work (engagement). However, there's a common misconception about happiness being a result of success. Many people think, "I'll be happy when I get that promotion," or "I'll feel great once I hit my sales target." The problem with this mindset is that as soon as you reach one goal, you're already setting the next one, which means the happiness you get from your success is always fleeting.

It turns out, it actually works the other way around: People who cultivate a positive mindset often perform better when they're up against a challenge. This is what I like to call the "happiness advantage" – the idea that almost every aspect of work improves when your brain is feeling positive. Rather than waiting for success to be happy, it seems that fostering a positive outlook can actually be a key factor in achieving success in the first place.

In 2015, the Journal of Labor Economics published the "Happiness and Productivity Experiment." This study investigated the link between happiness and productivity. Researchers created conditions to induce happiness in certain participants and then evaluated their productivity. The outcome was compelling: those who were made to feel happier showed significantly higher productivity compared to the control group. This experiment provided tangible evidence that a positive emotional state can indeed boost work performance, highlighting the practical benefits of fostering a positive work environment.

Positive Mindset and Relationships

It's pretty evident that people with a positive attitude tend to be more enjoyable company.

We all instinctively know that being around someone who smiles often, listens attentively, shows empathy, and can find the silver lining even in challenging situations makes for a more pleasant experience.

Studies are increasingly revealing that maintaining a positive outlook not only elevates our mood but also strengthens our relationships, leading to more meaningful and fulfilling interactions.

The interplay between a positive mental attitude and the quality of our relationships is profound. When we approach our interactions with optimism and positivity, we create an environment of trust, understanding, and mutual respect. This positive energy can help resolve conflicts more amicably, deepen connections, and foster a sense of closeness and security.

Research in the field of psychology has consistently shown that positive emotions are contagious. When one person in a relationship exhibits a positive attitude, it often spreads to the other person, enhancing the overall emotional tone of the interaction. This phenomenon is not just limited to romantic relationships but extends to friendships, familial bonds, and professional connections.

For example, a study published in the Journal of Personality and Social Psychology found that individuals who express genuine positive emotions are more likely to be perceived as supportive and caring by their partners. This perception, in turn, contributes to stronger and more resilient relationships. The study highlights how a positive disposition can act as a buffer during challenging times, helping partners navigate through difficulties with more ease and less stress.

Another interesting finding comes from a study in the field of organizational behavior. It suggests that a positive mindset in the workplace leads to better teamwork, improved communication, and increased job satisfaction. This indicates that positivity not only enhances personal relationships but also professional ones.

How to Cultivate a Positive Mindset

It's often thought that happiness is predominantly determined by our genes or environment, or a combination of both. While it's true that these factors do play a role, it's important to realize that our overall sense of well-being is quite flexible. The habits we form, our interactions with colleagues, and our perspective on stress are all aspects that we can control. By managing these areas of our lives, we can not only boost our happiness but also improve our health, relationships, and finance.

So, there are a myriad of reasons to cultivate a positive mindset. But how exactly can we do it? Let's explore.

Gratitude journals

A gratitude journal nurtures a positive and appreciative mindset. This practice involves regularly jotting down things for which you are thankful, fostering an atmosphere of gratitude in your daily life. The act of writing in a gratitude journal encourages a shift in focus - from what's lacking or problematic to what's abundant and positive. It's about acknowledging the small joys and victories, the warmth of a friend's support, the serenity of a quiet morning, or the satisfaction of a job well done.

This practice has deeper psychological benefits as well. It trains the mind to seek out and recognize the good, even in challenging circumstances. Over time, this nurtures an overall sense of well-being and happiness. It's not just about being thankful for the big, life-changing moments, but also about finding value and joy in the everyday - a delicious meal, a good book, a productive day at work, or a relaxing walk.

Additionally, gratitude journaling can improve mental health by reducing stress and anxiety. It shifts your attention away from stressors and towards what brings you peace and happiness. This habit also enhances self-awareness as you reflect on your experiences and feelings.

Mind Your Words

Language shapes not just how we communicate but also how we perceive and experience our lives. The choice of words, especially when describing our daily lives and emotions, has a profound impact. For example, using words like "boring," "busy," "angry," or "difficult" tends to cast a negative shadow on our experiences, influencing us to view our lives through a lens of negativity and dissatisfaction.

Conversely, adopting a vocabulary filled with words like "fun," "challenging," "simple," "engaging," "lively," and "interesting" can dramatically alter our perspective. This positive framing encourages us to see even mundane or challenging situations as opportunities for growth and enjoyment. It's a subtle yet powerful shift from enduring life to embracing it.

Take the common phrases "I have to go to work" or "I have to visit my parents." These sentences, laden with obligation, can make these activities feel burdensome. However, a simple switch to "I get to go to work" or "I get to see my parents" transforms these tasks into privileges, emphasizing gratitude and positivity.

This change in language does more than just alter perception; it can also lead to changes in behavior. When we start to see our daily tasks as opportunities or blessings, we approach them with more enthusiasm and a lighter heart. This shift can lead to a happier, more stress-free existence. By mindfully choosing our words, we're not just speaking differently; we're actively shaping a more positive reality for ourselves.

Breathing Exercises

Breathing exercises involve consciously controlling and regulating your breath, a process that directly influences the nervous system. For instance, deep diaphragmatic breathing, where you focus on filling your lungs completely and exhaling slowly, helps activate the parasympathetic nervous system. This activation triggers a relaxation response, reducing the body's stress response, and promoting a sense of calm and well-being.

There are various techniques tailored to different needs. For example, the 4-7-8 breathing technique, developed by Dr. Andrew Weil, involves inhaling for four seconds, holding the breath for seven seconds, and exhaling for eight seconds. This method is particularly effective for reducing anxiety and helping with sleep.

Another popular method is alternate nostril breathing, often used in yoga. It involves closing one nostril while inhaling through the other, and then switching nostrils for the exhale. This practice is known to balance the left and right hemispheres of the brain, enhancing mental clarity and emotional balance.

Regular practice of these breathing exercises can lead to improved emotional regulation, heightened focus, and a more positive and resilient mindset. By turning to these techniques during moments of stress or negativity, individuals can effectively shift their emotional state, fostering a more optimistic and serene outlook on life. This makes breathing exercises not just a tool for immediate stress relief, but also a daily practice for long-term emotional and mental well-being.

Mindfulness

Imagine navigating your day with a serene, keenly observant presence, where each moment is experienced fully, and every sensation and thought is acknowledged without judgment. This is the essence of mindfulness. Rooted in ancient practices, mindfulness involves bringing your complete attention to the present, observing your thoughts, feelings, bodily sensations, and the environment around you with a gentle, open mind.

Practicing mindfulness can transform how you engage with the world. It's often associated with meditation, where you might focus on your breath or the sensations in your body, allowing thoughts to come and go without getting caught up in them. But mindfulness extends beyond formal meditation; it's about maintaining this quality of conscious presence in all daily activities, whether eating, walking, or listening to someone.

Regular mindfulness practice offers profound benefits. It's been shown to reduce stress and anxiety, improve focus and cognitive flexibility, and enhance emotional regulation. It can deepen your connection to your experiences, creating a greater sense of harmony and appreciation for the present moment. By training your mind to be fully present, you cultivate a space where calmness and clarity can flourish, even amidst the chaos of everyday life. This mindful approach to living can lead to a richer, more fulfilling experience, marked by a deeper understanding of yourself and a more compassionate connection with others.

Positive Affirmation

Positive affirmations are short, powerful statements that, when repeated consistently, can have a profound impact on your mindset and overall outlook on life. They are designed to challenge and overcome negative and self-sabotaging thoughts, replacing them with empowering beliefs.

For some, it might be a bit corny at first (the way practising speech in a mirror is), but if you can push through the embarrassment, it is highly effective.

1. Self-Empowerment: "I am capable of overcoming any challenges that come my way." This affirmation instills a sense of strength and resilience.

2. Success Mindset: "I possess the qualities needed to be extremely successful." It fosters a belief in one's own abilities and potential for success.

3. Positivity and Prosperity: "My thoughts are filled with positivity and my life is plentiful with prosperity." This statement encourages an optimistic outlook and a mindset of abundance.

4. Embracing Change: "Today, I abandon my old habits and take up new, more positive ones." It focuses on personal growth and the ability to change for the better.

5. Self-Worth: "I am deserving of happiness, love, peace, freedom, money, and anything else I desire." This reinforces the idea that you are worthy of all good things in life.

6. Confidence and Competence: "I am strong, confident, and skilled enough to handle whatever comes next." It builds self-confidence and trust in one's abilities.

7. Continuous Improvement: "Every day in every way, I am getting better and better." It promotes the concept of continuous personal development.

8. Holistic Well-Being: "My body is healthy; my mind is brilliant; my soul is tranquil." This affirmation supports the idea of overall well-being.

9. Self-Belief: "I believe in myself and my abilities." It's a powerful statement of self-confidence and self-assurance.

10. Positive Perspective on Challenges: "Challenges are opportunities to grow and improve." This transforms the view of challenges as growth opportunities rather than obstacles.

Affirmations should be spoken in the present tense, as if they are already true.

View Failures As Lessons

Think of failures as stepping stones, each one a precious opportunity for growth and self-improvement. When you don't pass an exam, it's not a cue for self-criticism or resentment towards your teacher or institution. It's a moment to reflect, understand, and learn. Similarly, making a mistake on a project isn't a testament to your professional inadequacy; it's a chance to enhance your skills and knowledge. Each error, each misstep is packed with hidden lessons. When you embrace this perspective, you transform setbacks into growth opportunities, enriching your journey with wisdom and resilience. This approach fosters a nurturing, positive environment for personal development, steering you away from negativity and towards a path of continuous learning and self-compassion.

You Don't Have to Control Everything

Letting go and accepting that not everything is within our control is a liberating aspect of a positive mindset. It's common to seek control as a way to combat insecurities. For instance, in managing a work project, you naturally want to ensure success and might feel compelled to oversee every detail. While it's reasonable to have a degree of control over your tasks, trying to take on everyone else's can lead to undue stress and negativity.

This need for control can even extend to frustration over things like the weather, which is completely beyond our control. The key is to focus on how we react to these situations. In relationships, whether with colleagues, friends, or partners, trusting others and allowing them room to manage their responsibilities is crucial. This trust not only eases your stress but also strengthens these relationships. A positive mindset isn't about controlling everything; it's about managing our reactions and interactions in a balanced and trusting way.

Be Kind

Acts of kindness not only brightens someone else's day but also boost your own happiness. Studies indicate that people who volunteer or give to charity often experience a lift in their mood.

Why not try an experiment with this idea? When you find yourself with some free time, say an afternoon, grab a coin and give it a flip. If it lands on heads, treat yourself to something nice, like a relaxing manicure. But if it's tails, turn your focus outward – do something beneficial for your community or someone else. You could, for instance, reach out with a call or a letter to an elderly person who might appreciate the company.

Pay attention to how you feel both during and after this activity, in the following hours and days. It's an interesting way to observe first-hand the impact of kindness and self-care on your overall mood and well-being.

...

Training your mind to be more positive can be as rewarding and effective as working out at the gym. Recent research into neuroplasticity, which is the brain's ability to change and adapt even in adulthood, shows that developing new habits can actually rewire your brain.

This idea comes to life in a fascinating study. In December 2008, just before a particularly tough tax season, a group of tax managers at KPMG in New York and New Jersey participated in a unique experiment. The aim was to see if simple daily exercises could boost their happiness. The participants were asked to choose one of five activities, each known to foster positive change:

1. List three things they were grateful for each day.

2. Write a positive message to someone in their social network.

3. Meditate at their desk for two minutes.

4. Exercise for 10 minutes.

5. Spend two minutes writing about the most meaningful experience of their previous 24 hours.

They performed their chosen activity every day for three weeks. After the training, the results were remarkable. The participants' overall sense of well-being, engagement, and mood improved significantly compared to a control group. This uplift in spirits wasn't fleeting; when checked four months later, the participants still reported higher levels of optimism and life satisfaction. Their scores on the life satisfaction scale, a strong predictor of productivity and happiness at work, had notably increased from 22.96 to 27.23 on a 35-point scale.

This study beautifully illustrates how a small, daily positive exercise can lead to lasting happiness, turning it into a regular, almost habitual part of life.

Before We Get Started…

Remember, mindfulness journaling is a personal practice, and these questions are meant to guide and inspire you. Feel free to adapt and modify them to suit your needs and preferences. Explore, reflect, and embrace the opportunity to deepen your self-awareness and cultivate a sense of inner peace.

Date ___ / ___ / ___: S M T W Th F S

I feel:
(please circle)

because   because   because   because   because

_____ _____ _____ _____ _____

_____ _____ _____ _____ _____

Today I Am Grateful For

1. _____

2. _____

3. _____

What could help transform today into a remarkable day?

Reflective Writing

What are some of the most effective techniques you have used to manage your anxiety and stress?

_____

_____

_____

_____

_____

_____

_____

_____

Which of the following is a strategy for cultivating a positive mindset?

a) Practicing gratitude
b) Surrounding yourself with negative people
c) Focusing on past mistakes
d) Dwelling on negative thoughts

All Are Correct - Choose The Response You Feel Is Most Important To Remember

Date ___ / ___ / ___: S   M   T   W   Th   F   S

I feel:
(please circle)

because   because   because   because   because
_____   _____   _____   _____   _____
_____   _____   _____   _____   _____

Today I Am Grateful For

1. _____
2. _____
3. _____

What could help transform today into a remarkable day?

Reflective Writing

How have you incorporated self-care into your
daily routine to help reduce stress and anxiety?

_____

_____

_____

_____

_____

_____

_____

What is the importance of self-talk in cultivating a positive mindset?

a) It helps to reinforce negative beliefs
b) It promotes self-doubt and negative thinking
c) It can shape your attitude and perception
d) It hinders personal growth and development

All Are Correct - Choose The Response You Feel Is Most Important To Remember

Date ___ / ___ / ___ : S M T W Th F S

I feel:
(please circle)

because _____ because _____ because _____ because _____ because _____

Today I Am Grateful For

1. _____
2. _____
3. _____

What could help transform today into a remarkable day?

Reflective Writing

What have you found to be the most effective tools to cope with anxiety and stress?

_____

_____

_____

_____

_____

_____

_____

How does setting realistic goals contribute to a positive mindset?

a) It leads to constant comparison with others
b) It creates pressure and stress if not achieved
c) It fosters a sense of accomplishment and motivation
d) It discourages personal growth and improvement

All Are Correct - Choose The Response You Feel Is Most Important To Remember

Date ___ / ___ / ___: S M T W Th F S

I feel:
(please circle)

because _____ because _____ because _____ because _____ because _____

Today I Am Grateful For

1. _____
2. _____
3. _____

What could help transform today into a remarkable day?

Reflective Writing

What has been the biggest challenge you have faced when managing your anxiety and stress?

_____

_____

_____

_____

_____

_____

_____

Why is it important to practice self-care when cultivating a positive mindset?

a) It distracts from personal growth and development
b) It promotes burnout and exhaustion
c) It helps maintain emotional and physical well-being
d) It leads to increased negative thoughts and self-talk

All Are Correct - Choose The Response You Feel Is Most Important To Remember

Date ___ / ___ / ___ : S   M   T   W   Th   F   S

I feel:
(please circle)

because _____   because _____   because _____   because _____   because _____

Today I Am Grateful For

1. _____
2. _____
3. _____

What could help transform today into a remarkable day?

Reflective Writing

What kind of balance have you found between recognizing your stress and anxiety and taking care of yourself?

_____

_____

_____

_____

_____

_____

_____

How does embracing failure contribute to a positive mindset?

a) It reinforces fear of taking risks
b) It promotes self-criticism and doubt
c) It encourages learning and personal growth
d) It discourages resilience and perseverance

All Are Correct - Choose The Response You Feel Is Most Important To Remember

Date ___ / ___ / ___ : S   M   T   W   Th   F   S

I feel:
(please circle)

because   because   because   because   because
_____ _____ _____ _____ _____
_____ _____ _____ _____ _____

Today I Am Grateful For

1. _____
2. _____
3. _____

What could help transform today into a remarkable day?

Reflective Writing

How has your relationship with stress and anxiety changed over time?

_____

_____

_____

_____

_____

_____

_____

_____

How can reframing negative situations contribute to a positive mindset?

a) It reinforces negative thought patterns
b) It maintains a victim mentality
c) It promotes optimism and resilience
d) It encourages dwelling on the negative

All Are Correct - Choose The Response You Feel Is Most Important To Remember

Date ___ / ___ / ___ : S M T W Th F S

I feel:
(please circle)

because _____ because _____ because _____ because _____ because _____
_____ _____ _____ _____ _____

Today I Am Grateful For

1. _____
2. _____
3. _____

What could help transform today into a remarkable day?

Reflective Writing

What strategies do you use to manage your stress
and anxiety in the moment?

_____

_____

_____

_____

_____

_____

_____

How does practicing mindfulness contribute to a positive mindset?

a)   It encourages rumination and overthinking

b)   It promotes being present and aware of the moment

c)   It leads to increased stress and anxiety

d)   It hinders personal growth and self-reflection

All Are Correct - Choose The Response You Feel Is Most Important To Remember

Date ___ / ___ / ___: S   M   T   W   Th   F   S

I feel:
(please circle)

because _____   because _____   because _____   because _____   because _____

Today I Am Grateful For

1. _____
2. _____
3. _____

What could help transform today into a remarkable day?

Reflective Writing

How have you been able to recognize when your stress or anxiety is becoming too much?

_____

_____

_____

_____

_____

_____

_____

Why is it important to surround yourself with positive people when cultivating a positive mindset?

a) They provide constant criticism and negativity
b) They can be a source of support and encouragement
c) They increase self-doubt and negative self-talk
d) They hinder personal growth and development

All Are Correct - Choose The Response You Feel Is Most Important To Remember

Date ___ / ___ / ___ : **S M T W Th F S**

I feel:
(please circle)

because because because because because

___ ___ ___ ___ ___

___ ___ ___ ___ ___

Today I Am Grateful For

1. _____
2. _____
3. _____

What could help transform today into a remarkable day?

Reflective Writing

What do you do when you find yourself
overwhelmed with anxiety and stress?

_____

_____

_____

_____

_____

_____

_____

How does practicing forgiveness contribute to a positive mindset?

a) It promotes holding grudges and resentment
b) It encourages self-pity and victim mentality
c) It fosters inner peace and emotional well-being
d) It leads to increased anger and bitterness

All Are Correct - Choose The Response You Feel Is Most Important To Remember

Date ___ / ___ / ___ : S M T W Th F S

I feel:
(please circle)

because _____ because _____ because _____ because _____ because _____
_____ _____ _____ _____ _____

Today I Am Grateful For
1. _____
2. _____
3. _____

What could help transform today into a remarkable day?

Reflective Writing

What have been some of the biggest successes you
have had in managing your stress and anxiety?

_____

_____

_____

_____

_____

_____

_____

How does focusing on the present moment contribute to a positive mindset?

a) It leads to constant worry and anxiety about the future
b) It promotes regret and dwelling on the past
c) It fosters gratitude and appreciation for the present
d) It encourages negative thoughts and self-talk

All Are Correct - Choose The Response You Feel Is Most Important To Remember

Date ___ / ___ / ___ : S   M   T   W   Th   F   S

I feel:
(please circle)

because   because   because   because   because
_____   _____   _____   _____   _____
_____   _____   _____   _____   _____

Today I Am Grateful For

1. _____
2. _____
3. _____

What could help transform today into a remarkable day?

Reflective Writing

What advice would you give to someone who is trying to manage their stress and anxiety?

_____

_____

_____

_____

_____

_____

_____

How does adopting a growth mindset contribute to cultivating a positive mindset?

a) It reinforces self-limiting beliefs and thoughts
b) It promotes a fixed mindset and resistance to change
c) It encourages resilience and a belief in personal improvement
d) It leads to increased self-doubt and negative self-talk

All Are Correct - Choose The Response You Feel Is Most Important To Remember

Date ___ / ___ / ___: S   M   T   W   Th   F   S

I feel:
(please circle)

because   because   because   because   because
_____   _____   _____   _____   _____
_____   _____   _____   _____   _____

Today I Am Grateful For

1. _____
2. _____
3. _____

What could help transform today into a remarkable day?

Reflective Writing

How has learning about stress and anxiety
management helped you in your daily life?

_____

_____

_____

_____

_____

_____

_____

How does practicing kindness and compassion towards oneself contribute to a positive mindset?

a) It reinforces self-criticism and self-judgment
b) It promotes self-love and self-acceptance
c) It leads to increased comparison with others
d) It hinders personal growth and development

All Are Correct - Choose The Response You Feel Is Most Important To Remember

Date ___ / ___ / ___ : S   M   T   W   Th   F   S

I feel:
(please circle)

because   because   because   because   because

_____   _____   _____   _____   _____
_____   _____   _____   _____   _____

Today I Am Grateful For

1. _____
2. _____
3. _____

What could help transform today into a remarkable day?

Reflective Writing
How have you been able to stay motivated to effectively manage your stress and anxiety?

_____

_____

_____

_____

_____

_____

_____

_____

How does practicing gratitude contribute to a positive mindset?

a) It fosters negativity and discontent
b) It promotes a victim mentality and self-pity
c) It encourages a sense of contentment and happiness
d) It leads to increased self-doubt and negative self-talk

All Are Correct - Choose The Response You Feel Is Most Important To Remember

Date ___ / ___ / ___: S   M   T   W   Th   F   S

I feel:
(please circle)

because   because   because   because   because

_____ _____ _____ _____ _____

_____ _____ _____ _____ _____

Today I Am Grateful For

1. _____
2. _____
3. _____

What could help transform today into a remarkable day?

Reflective Writing

What changes have you made to your lifestyle to help reduce stress and anxiety?

_____

_____

_____

_____

_____

_____

_____

How does embracing a healthy lifestyle contribute to a positive mindset?

a) It promotes excessive stress and busy-ness
b) It reinforces unhealthy habits and mindset
c) It fosters physical and mental well-being
d) It leads to increased negative thoughts and self-talk

All Are Correct - Choose The Response You Feel Is Most Important To Remember

Date __ / __ / __: S   M   T   W   Th   F   S

I feel:
(please circle)

because   because   because   because   because
_____   _____   _____   _____   _____
_____   _____   _____   _____   _____

Today I Am Grateful For

1. _____
2. _____
3. _____

What could help transform today into a remarkable day?

Reflective Writing

What resources have been the most helpful to you
in managing your stress and anxiety?

_____

_____

_____

_____

_____

_____

_____

How does seeking personal growth and learning contribute to a positive mindset?

a) It reinforces self-limiting beliefs and thoughts
b) It promotes stagnation and resistance to change
c) It encourages self-improvement and a belief in one's potential
d) It leads to increased self-doubt and negative self-talk

All Are Correct - Choose The Response You Feel Is Most Important To Remember

As we reach the final pages of this journey through "Positive Mindset," I want to extend my heartfelt thanks to you. Your commitment to exploring positivity and its transformative power is not only commendable but a testament to your desire for personal growth and a richer, more fulfilling life experience.

Remember, the journey towards a positive mindset is ongoing and ever-evolving. Each day presents new opportunities to apply these principles, to learn, and to grow. I encourage you to revisit these pages whenever you need a reminder of your incredible potential to foster positivity and resilience in the face of life's challenges.

As we part ways, I leave you with a quote that has been a guiding star in my journey: "The greatest discovery of any generation is that a human can alter his life by altering his attitude."

– William James.

Thank you for allowing me to be a part of your journey. May your path be filled with light, hope, and endless possibilities. Farewell, and may you carry the spirit of positivity with you, today and always.

With gratitude and best wishes,

Sensei Paul David

Reflective Writing

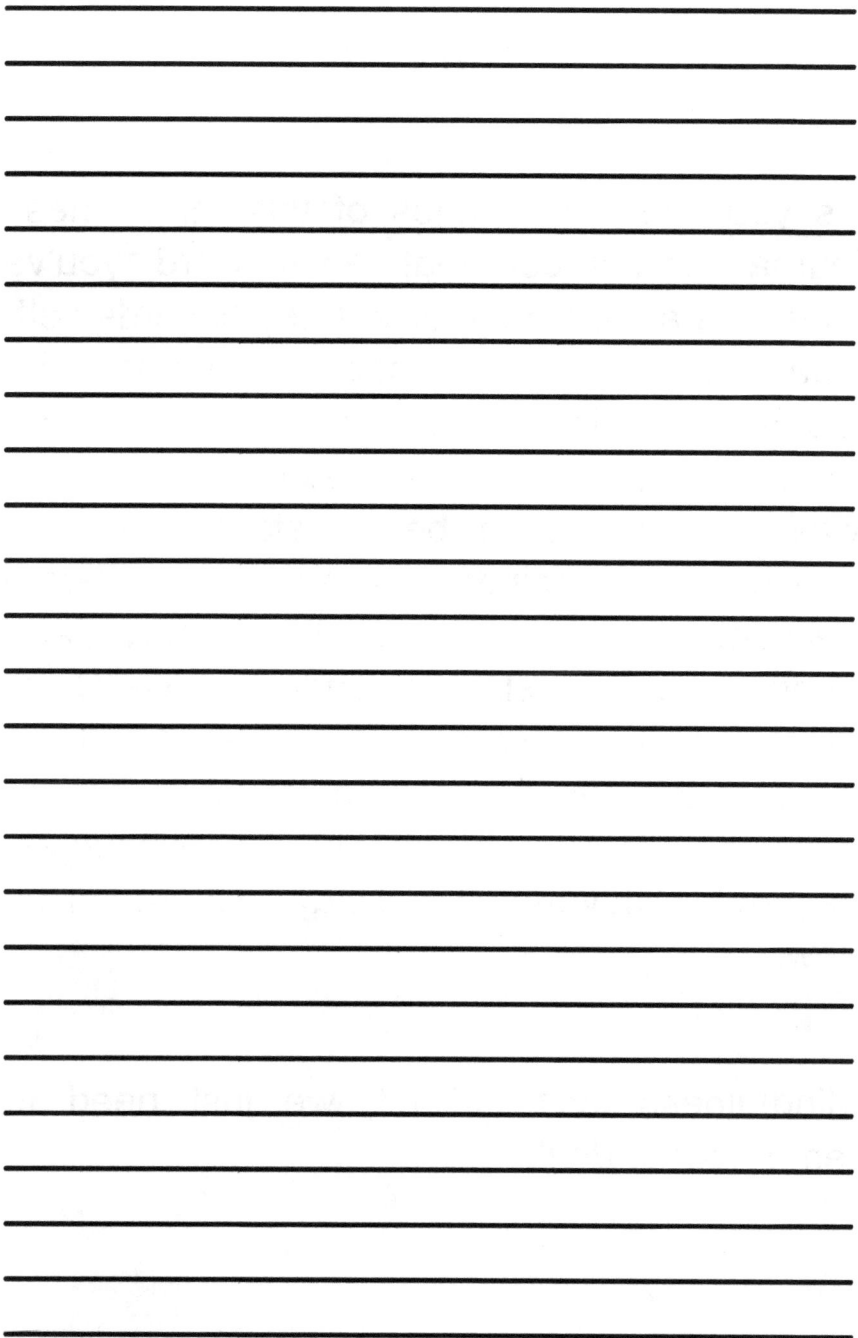

The End

As you close the pages of this mindfulness journal, remember that each word you've written is a step on your journey towards self-awareness and inner peace. Embrace the moments of clarity, the revelations, and even the uncertainties you've encountered along the way. Let this journal be a testament to your growth and a reminder that every day offers a new opportunity to be present, to observe, and to appreciate the simple wonders of life. Carry these lessons forward, and may your path be filled with mindful moments and serene reflections. Until we meet again in these pages, be gentle with yourself and stay anchored in the now.

Mindfulness isn't difficult, we just need to remember to do it.

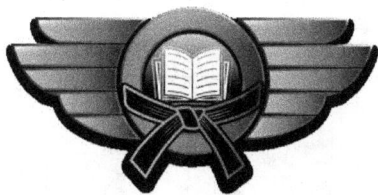

Thank You!

If you found this book helpful, I would be grateful if you would **post an honest review on Amazon** so this book can reach other supportive readers like you!

All you need to do is digitally flip to the back and leave your review. Or visit amazon.com/author/senseipauldavid click the correct book cover and click on the blue link next to the yellow stars that say, "customer reviews."

As always...
It's a great day to be alive!

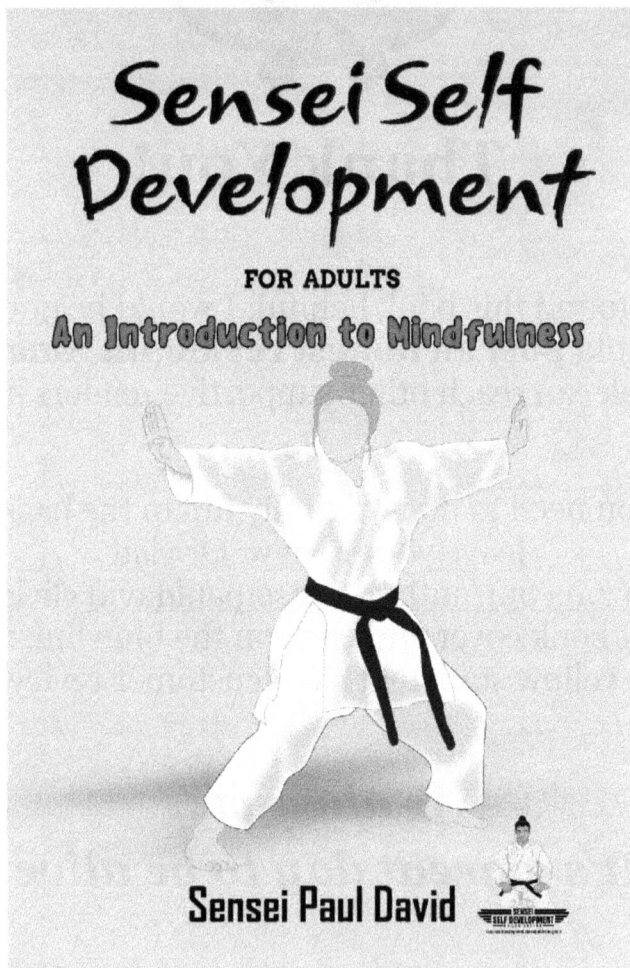

Sensei Self Development

FOR ADULTS

An Introduction to Mindfulness

Sensei Paul David

Check Out The SSD Chronicles Series CLICK HERE

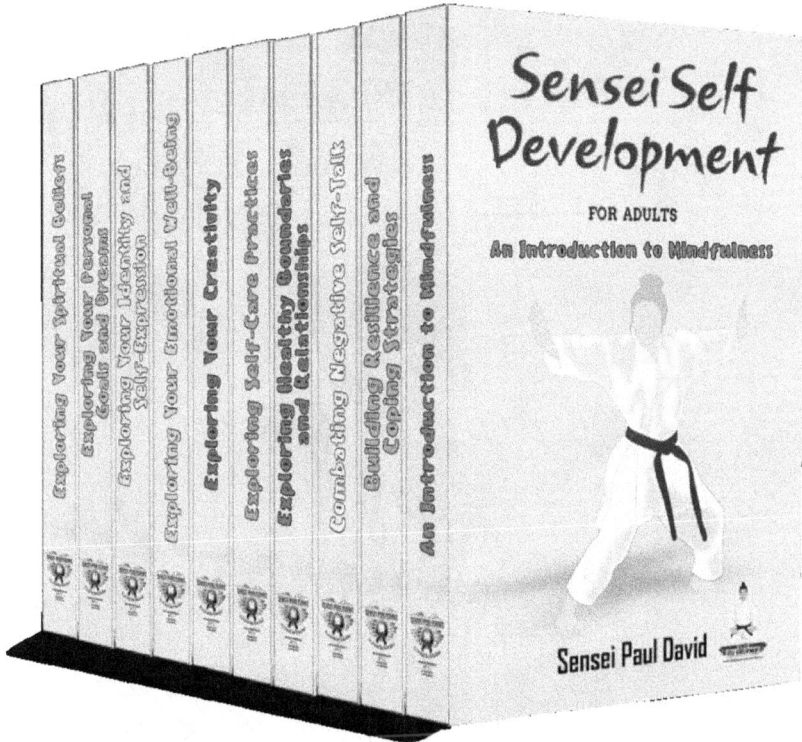

Sensei Self Development

FOR ADULTS

An Introduction to Mindfulness

Sensei Paul David

Exploring Your Spiritual Beliefs

Exploring Your Personal Goals and Dreams

Exploring Your Identity and Self-Expression

Exploring Your Emotional Well-Being

Exploring Your Creativity

Exploring Self-Care Practices

Exploring Healthy Boundaries and Relationships

Combatting Negative Self-Talk

Building Resilience and Coping Strategies

An Introduction to Mindfulness

Get/Share Your FREE All-Ages Mental Health eBook Now at

www.senseiselfdevelopment.com

Or CLICK HERE

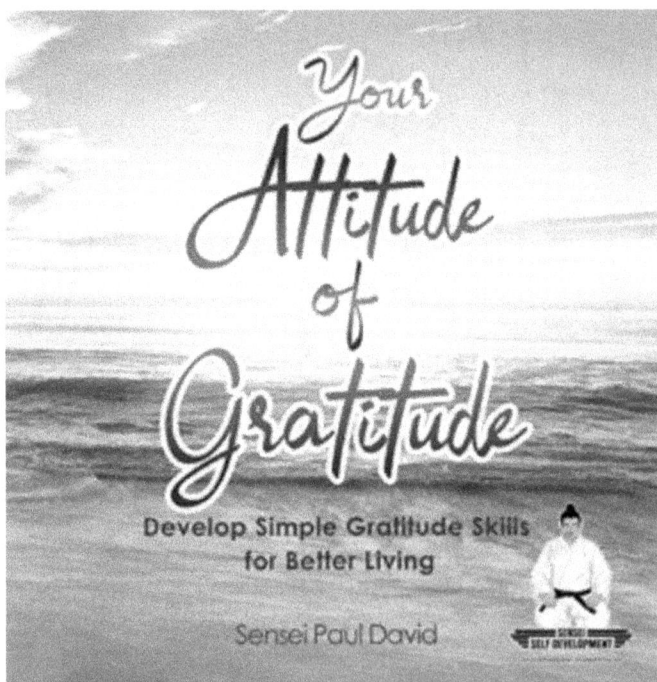

senseiselfdevelopment.com

Click Another Book In The SSD BOOK SERIES:

senseipublishing.com/SSD_SERIES

CLICK HERE

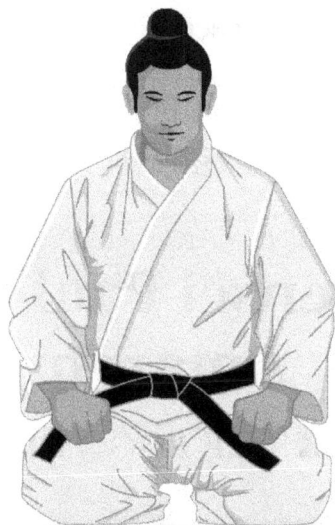

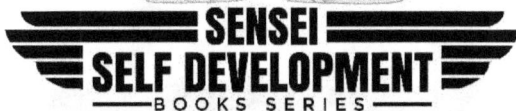

SENSEI
SELF DEVELOPMENT
— BOOKS SERIES —
senseiselfdevelopment.senseipublishing.com

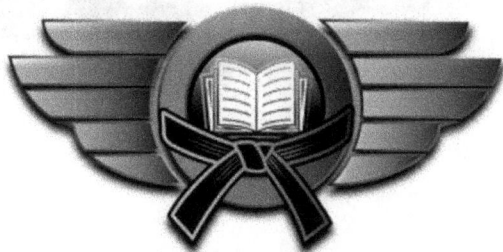

Join Our Publishing Journey!

If you would like to receive FREE BOOKS, please visit **www.senseipublishing.com**. Join our newsletter by entering your email address in the pop-up box

Follow Sensei Paul David on Amazon

CLICK THE LOGO BELOW

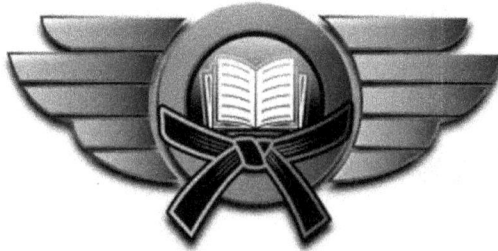

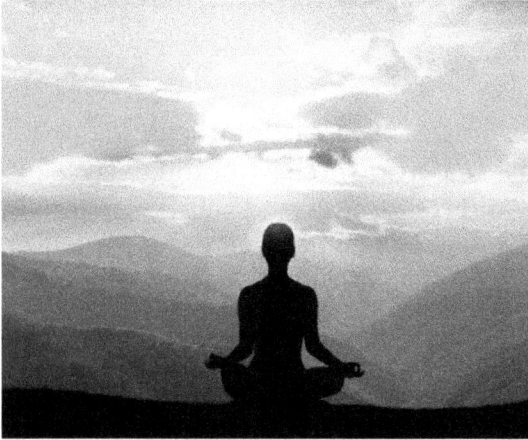

FREE BONUS!!!
Experience Over 25 FREE Engaging Guided Meditations!

Prized Skills & Practices for Adults & Kids. Help Restore Deep-Sleep, Lower Stress, Improve Posture, Navigate Uncertainty & More.

Download the Free Insight Timer App and click the link below:
http://insig.ht/sensei_paul

About Sensei Publishing

Sensei Publishing commits itself to helping people of all ages transform into better versions of themselves by providing high-quality and research-based self-development books with an emphasis on mental health and guided meditations. Sensei Publishing offers well-written e-books, audiobooks, paperbacks and online courses that simplify complicated but practical topics in line with its mission to inspire people towards positive transformation.

It's a great day to be alive!

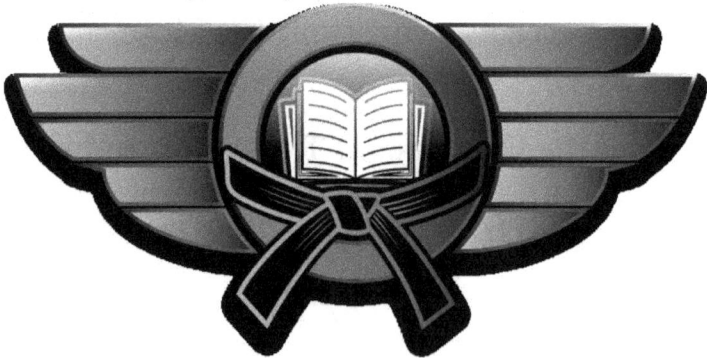

About the Author

I create simple & transformative eBooks & Guided Meditations for Adults & Children proven to help navigate uncertainty, solve niche problems & bring families closer together.

I'm a former finance project manager, private pilot, jiu-jitsu instructor, musician & former University of Toronto Fitness Trainer. I prefer a science-based approach to focus on these & other areas in my life to stay humble & hungry to evolve. I hope you enjoy my work and I'd love to hear your feedback.

- It's a great day to be alive!

Sensei Paul David

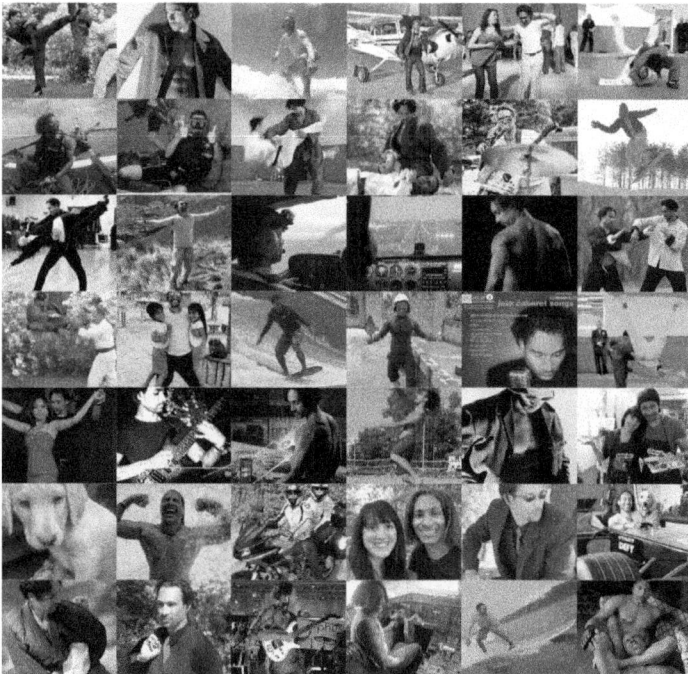

Scan & Follow/Like/Subscribe: Facebook, Instagram,
YouTube: @senseipublishing

Scan using your phone/iPad camera for Social Media
Visit us at www.senseipublishing.com and sign up for our
newsletter to learn more about our exciting books and to
experience our FREE Guided Meditations for Kids & Adults.

www.ingramcontent.com/pod-product-compliance
Lightning Source LLC
Chambersburg PA
CBHW071244020426

42333CB00015B/1612